Genital Herpes

A Beginner's 3-Step Guide for Women on Managing Genital Herpes Through Diet, With Sample Recipes

mf

copyright © 2022 Mary Golanna

All rights reserved No part of this book may be reproduced, or stored in a retrieval system, or transmitted in any form or by any means, electronic, mechanical, photocopying, recording, or otherwise, without express written permission of the publisher.

Disclaimer

By reading this disclaimer, you are accepting the terms of the disclaimer in full. If you disagree with this disclaimer, please do not read the guide.

All of the content within this guide is provided for informational and educational purposes only, and should not be accepted as independent medical or other professional advice. The author is not a doctor, physician, nurse, mental health provider, or registered nutritionist/dietician. Therefore, using and reading this guide does not establish any form of a physician-patient relationship.

Always consult with a physician or another qualified health provider with any issues or questions you might have regarding any sort of medical condition. Do not ever disregard any qualified professional medical advice or delay seeking that advice because of anything you have read in this guide. The information in this guide is not intended to be any sort of medical advice and should not be used in lieu of any medical advice by a licensed and qualified medical professional.

The information in this guide has been compiled from a variety of known sources. However, the author cannot attest to or guarantee the accuracy of each source and thus should not be held liable for any errors or omissions.

You acknowledge that the publisher of this guide will not be held liable for any loss or damage of any kind incurred as a result of this guide or the reliance on any information provided within this guide. You acknowledge and agree that you assume all risk and responsibility for any action you undertake in response to the information in this guide.

Using this guide does not guarantee any particular result (e.g., weight loss or a cure). By reading this guide, you acknowledge that there are no guarantees to any specific outcome or results you can expect.

All product names, diet plans, or names used in this guide are for identification purposes only and are the property of their respective owners. The use of these names does not imply endorsement. All other trademarks cited herein are the property of their respective owners.

Where applicable, this guide is not intended to be a substitute for the original work of this diet plan and is, at most, a supplement to the original work for this diet plan and never a direct substitute. This guide is a personal expression of the facts of that diet plan.

Where applicable, persons shown in the cover images are stock photography models and the publisher has obtained the rights to use the images through license agreements with third-party stock image companies.

Table of Contents

Introduction — 7
What Is Genital Herpes? — 9
   Symptoms — 9
   Causes — 10
   Risk Factors — 10
What Women Should Know About Genital Herpes — 12
   Hormonal influence — 12
   Antiviral medication is safe during pregnancy — 13
   After giving birth, a mother can give herpes to her baby. — 13
Diagnosis, Management, and Treatment — 15
   Diagnosis — 15
   Management and Treatment — 16
   Herbs and Supplements to Try — 17
   Prevention — 18
Managing Genital Herpes with Diet — 20
A 3-Step Plan for Managing Genital Herpes — 23
   Step 1: Start cutting out trigger foods — 23
   Step 2: Focus on Filling Your Diet with Those Foods Listed Above — 24
   Step 3: Manage Your Stress — 24
Sample Recipes — 26
   Asparagus and Greens Salad with Tahini and Poppy Seed Dressing — 27
   Cauliflower and Mushroom Bake — 28
   Lemon Roasted Broccoli — 29
   Mixed Vegetable Roast with Lemon Zest — 30
   Roasted Veggies — 31
   Stir Fry Broccoli, Onions, and Carrots — 32
   Healthy Vegetable Bowl — 33

Veggie Bowl	35
Healthy Zucchini Fries	39
Avocado and Caesar Salad	41
Cobb Salad	42
Salmon and Asparagus	44
Lemon-Baked Salmon	45
Baked Salmon	47
Salmon Filet with Lemon and Garlic	49
Roasted Broccoli and Salmon	51
Smoked Salmon and Baked Eggs in Avocado	53
Tuna and Veggies Wrap	54
Conclusion	**55**
References and Helpful Links	**56**

Introduction

Genital herpes infection is caused by one of the two types of herpes simplex virus or HSV. In the United States, there are about 45 million Americans who have herpes infections. American women fall under 20-25% of this population, or about 1 out of 5 women have this infection.

Herpes symptoms include painful blisters on the genitals or mouth. Herpes can be managed but not cured by taking antiviral medications and/or using natural herbs and supplements that help regulate the immune system. However, managing herpes can be hard to do if you're eating a diet high in processed foods and sugars. Most Americans eat this type of diet that feeds the growth of herpes-causing viruses in their bodies.

This beginner's quick start guide offers practical tools for women who want to manage their herpes through diet by regulating the immune system, while also reducing recurrences. Through diet and lifestyle changes, women can help reduce the frequency and severity of herpes recurrences. The guide includes information on how to successfully manage genital herpes through diet with sample meal plans and recipes.

In this guide, you will discover...

- What genital herpes is and how women contract it
- Typical symptoms of genital herpes
- The risk factors associated with contracting herpes
- The connection between food and immunity
- What foods to avoid and what foods to include for managing genital herpes
- Sample recipes

What Is Genital Herpes?

Genital herpes infection is caused by one of the two types of herpes simplex virus or HSV. Type 2 HSV causes about 90 to 95% of genital herpes infections and is typically contracted through sexual contact, while type 1 HSV causes about 60 to 70% of oral herpes infections and is most often contracted in childhood through non-sexual contact.

Symptoms

Herpes symptoms include painful blisters on the genitals or mouth. Symptoms can show up within 2 weeks of contracting herpes and then recur an average of 4 to 5 times a year, with each episode lasting approximately 7 days at a time.

A major outbreak can produce sores that cover all areas from the waist down and cause flu-like symptoms such as fever, swollen glands, and body aches. Herpes outbreaks make some women more susceptible to infection by HIV/AIDS and other STDs (sexually transmitted diseases), according to the World Health Organization (WHO).

In addition, people may experience scabs ulcers, itching, burning, and painful urination with herpes.

Causes

There are two types of herpes simplex virus that cause genital herpes: HSV-1 and HSV-2. Both can infect the genitals through oral sex, but only HSV-1 usually causes sores in the mouth. However, both viruses can be found in either region throughout their active periods. Some people experience very mild symptoms or none at all, while others may also have swelling of lymph glands along with blisters and pain.

The first infection with any one type of HSV creates antibodies to fight it off completely; however, future outbreaks (no matter which strain of HSV is causing them) tend to be less severe than the first outbreak because your body has already formed its protection against the strain of herpes you are carrying. If you have contracted type 1 HSV, it is not possible to contract type 2.

Risk Factors

People who suffer from chronic stress are more likely to contract herpes because stress suppresses the immune system, which makes it harder for your body to fight off an HSV infection. Other factors that can lead to contracting genital herpes include:

- Older age since the immune system weakens with age and becomes less adequate in fending off the herpes virus.
- Weak immune systems: People who have acquired immunodeficiency syndrome (AIDS), children, and the elderly are more susceptible to acquiring HSV infection than healthy adults. Some people may also reduce their risk of contracting herpes if they strengthen their immune systems.

What Women Should Know About Genital Herpes

Genital herpes is a chronic lifelong infection that can be managed but not cured. About 20%-25% of American women have herpes, although around 80%-90% are unaware they have it because there are often no symptoms present. That means the majority of women have not been tested for herpes even though they are at risk of contracting the virus.

Hormonal influence

Women often contract herpes during pregnancy, when their immune systems are suppressed by pregnancy hormones that prevent an active immune response against the herpes virus. This means that instead of immediately attacking and destroying the virus, pregnant women's bodies allow the herpes virus to remain dormant in the body for years before recurring as a genital outbreak. This recurrence can happen during pregnancy or any time that hormonal levels drops, such as during menstruation and menopause.

Antiviral medication is safe during pregnancy

Today doctors know that the antiviral medications used to treat genital herpes during pregnancy are both safe and effective. The CDC (Centers for Disease Control & Prevention) states, "the risk of having an asymptomatic herpes outbreak as a pregnant woman is much smaller than previously believed." The CDC advises the following:

Women with herpes should take steps to protect their babies from infection.

If you have genital herpes and have vaginal or anal intercourse at any time during pregnancy, you are at risk of passing the virus to your baby. In this case, get a doctor's help in reducing possible complications from an outbreak before birth. Because of the risk of infection during birth, doctors may perform a "C-section" (cesarean section) to reduce the chance that the baby will be exposed to herpes.

After giving birth, a mother can give herpes to her baby.

Herpes is spread from the mother's genital area to the baby during vaginal delivery as the baby passes through the birth canal. In rare cases, if a woman has an active infection around the time of delivery, doctors may recommend a C-section to reduce possible complications from herpes.

However, many women with herpes may give birth normally, while some babies contract the virus from a cesarean delivery.

A woman who has active genital herpes near the time of delivery may want to warn anyone taking care of her baby about the risk of infection.

For most women, genital herpes doesn't cause other serious health problems.

Studies of pregnant women with herpes have found that for most, it's a minor infection that does not pose serious health problems.

Diagnosis, Management, and Treatment

Diagnosis

You can be diagnosed with herpes by taking a swab culture test of the blisters or sores. Most pregnant women are tested for herpes during their first prenatal visit, according to the CDC (Centers for Disease Control and Prevention). However, if you experience your first outbreak during pregnancy, tell your doctor immediately so that your baby is not at risk of contracting herpes through birth. There is no test for herpes during birth, so be sure to tell your doctor if you have had an outbreak recently.

Besides swab culture tests, there are PCR tests. PCR refers to "polymerase chain reaction," a method of multiplying very small amounts of DNA so it can be analyzed. A PCR test is used for women who experience an active herpes outbreak during labor or delivery because these tests are 95%-99% accurate in detecting maternal herpes infection.

Another method is through a blood test, which can be taken at the doctor's office and takes only about 30 minutes to complete.

The CDC recommends all pregnant women who have never had genital herpes be tested once during their pregnancy.

Management and Treatment

Unfortunately, there is currently no cure for herpes, but there are many medications that can be used to treat it. According to the CDC (Centers for Disease Control and Prevention) oral antiviral medications such as acyclovir, valacyclovir and famciclovir may be prescribed during pregnancy when you experience your first herpes outbreak to prevent the spread to your baby. Talk to your medical provider about what medication is right for you, and how much time you will need off work or school.

You can manage genital herpes by seeking out proper medical treatment and taking care of yourself so that your immune system is strong. This will decrease the painful symptoms of an outbreak.

Since outbreaks are more frequent during the first 6 months after infection, you should drink plenty of fluids to prevent dehydration and avoid constipation, which can make herpes sores worse. If you experience an outbreak, it's best to take simple, gentle baths. It may also help to apply aloe vera gel or use a cool compress. Be sure not to rub or scrub the area and wear loose clothing whenever possible.

Also, some prescription antiviral medications can be taken daily to reduce the number of herpes outbreaks. The CDC also claims that daily suppressive therapy for herpes has been shown to decrease the risk of transmission from a person with herpes who is already infected, to a partner.

When seeking treatment it's important to find a medical professional you trust and feel comfortable with. If you have herpes, treatment for it should be discussed with your doctor or OBGYN. Discussing treatment early on can help reduce the number of outbreaks you experience in the future.

Finally, there are some alternative ways to manage herpes. You can take zinc, lysine, or vitamin C supplements to help reduce the number of future outbreaks. There are also some types of botanical remedies that may help, although they have not been proven in clinical settings.

Herbs and Supplements to Try

There are several herbs and supplements that have been suggested for use in herpes treatment. These include lysine, quercetin, licorice root extract, propolis, arginine, olive leaf extract, bergamot oil, echinacea Angustifolia herb tincture, or tea formula. Consult your doctor before trying any of these remedies.

Additionally, you might try acupressure for relief from your symptoms. Creating pressure on certain points in your hands and feet has helped some women feel less pain during an outbreak. Finally, acupuncture may be helpful, with some studies showing it helped reduce the number of outbreaks women experienced.

Be sure to speak with your doctor before trying any alternative treatments for herpes, especially since they can have negative interactions with prescription medications you may be taking for genital herpes. Seeking treatment from a medical professional is the best way to manage your condition and relieve pain in future outbreaks.

Prevention

The best way to prevent herpes outbreaks is by avoiding sex when sores or other symptoms are present and using condoms for all types of sexual intercourse. Condoms can reduce the risk of transmitting herpes even when symptoms aren't present.

If you have herpes, avoiding sex during outbreaks is important to prevent the spread of it to your partner. You or your partner may also wish to avoid oral or anal sex if sores are present in those areas. Take care not to share personal items such as towels, clothing, or eating utensils.

You can take steps to lower your risk of transmitting herpes during sex, especially when your partner doesn't have the virus. Using a condom correctly every time you have oral, vaginal, or anal sex can help reduce your chances of giving your partner genital herpes. Avoiding sex when sores are present is another way to protect your partner.

People with herpes tend to have fewer outbreaks over time. This doesn't mean that the virus is completely gone, but it does mean that you're taking better care of yourself and helping suppress the virus. Symptoms may come back from time to time, perhaps when you're sick or under stress, but it's important to remember that they'll disappear again.

Managing Genital Herpes with Diet

Diet is an important part of managing any medical condition, and that's no different when it comes to herpes.

Your diet can have a big impact on how often you have outbreaks, so eating a healthy diet with plenty of fresh fruits and vegetables is a great place to start. Your doctor or OBGYN may also suggest taking vitamin supplements as part of your treatment plan.

There is a connection between what foods you eat and outbreaks of herpes. Some foods seem to be particularly effective at keeping outbreaks under control, while others can trigger an outbreak or make it worse. Studies show that eating plenty of whole grains and fish can help reduce herpes outbreaks, while eating processed foods and refined carbs like white bread and sugar may trigger them.

Choosing the right foods for your genital herpes diet might seem complicated at first, but once you get started it will be easy to find out which types of food work best for you.

There are several types of foods you need to avoid:

- Alcohol is a diuretic and can dehydrate you. It may also cause or worsen irritable bowel syndrome (IBS) in some people, making herpes symptoms worse. Some studies have also shown that drinking alcohol may increase the risk of herpes transmission from a person who has herpes to a sex partner. It's a good idea to avoid drinking alcohol when in a relationship, especially if you or your partner has herpes.
- Sugary foods are high in calories but don't provide any nutritional value to your body. They can prolong outbreaks by upsetting your blood sugar levels
- It's important to remember that everyone with herpes should avoid caffeine as much as possible since it can make outbreaks worse. This means cutting down on coffee and other caffeinated drinks.
- Foods high in Arginine may also give you or your partner a tingling sensation around the genitals. Arginine is a natural amino acid that helps cells grow and may trigger outbreaks in people with herpes. Some foods that have arginine include chocolate, nuts, and lentils. In contrast, lysine may help reduce the number of outbreaks you or your partner experience. Lysine is another amino acid that binds to arginine and helps stop it from entering cells, including herpes-infected ones. Foods high in lysine include fruits like apples, pears, and fish.

Here are some foods to eat:

- Healthy fats, such as omega-3 fatty acids, help reduce your risk for heart disease and depression. Healthy fats also play a role in helping your body absorb vitamin D. This includes salmon and avocados.
- Vitamin C is needed for the growth, function, and repair of all body tissues. This is especially true of connective tissue like collagen, which is found inside the walls of your blood vessels. Increasing vitamin C in your diet may also help reduce the risk of cold sores forming on your lips or around your mouth during stress. This includes some foods such as broccoli and bell peppers.
- Zinc helps to create new cells and repair damage, so it's important for the production of white blood cells too. This includes oysters and other seafood.
- Vitamin E is a powerful antioxidant that may help reduce your risk of having an outbreak. An example would be spinach.
- Vitamin A is another antioxidant that can help your body fight off infection. Foods high in vitamin A include sweet potatoes, carrots, and peas

A 3-Step Plan for Managing Genital Herpes

Now that you have learned about genital herpes and how to eat for better overall health, you can put what you've learned into action with the following 3-step plan.

Step 1: Start cutting out trigger foods

The first step is to get rid of all the foods that you may be sensitive to and replace them with healthy alternatives. You'll be on your way to a better lifestyle and longer-lasting health in no time. This means cutting out foods like sodas, processed snacks, and pizza. If you are on medication for your herpes, it's important to talk to your doctor before making any dietary changes.

Grab a bag and throw away any food that you think might be causing or triggering outbreaks. If it doesn't go into the right bin, then toss it out.

Step 2: Focus on Filling Your Diet with Those Foods Listed Above

The next step is to stock your kitchen or pantry with healthy foods that you can eat daily. You'll notice that many of the suggested foods above are nutrient-rich and provide you with an abundance of vitamins, minerals, and antioxidants. This includes lots of fresh fruits, vegetables, healthy fats like avocados, olive oil, flaxseed oil, and lean meats such as fish.

When you're at the grocery store or farmer's market, stay away from the middle of the store. This is where you'll find processed foods that are packed with additives, sodium, sugars, and saturated fat. Remember to eat more produce so your body gets all the vitamins it needs.

You now know which foods to eat, but when should you have them? It's best not to have any food within 2 hours before or after taking herpes medication since this will reduce its effectiveness. For example, if you take Valacyclovir 1 hour before eating a meal, then skip having any food for at least 1 hour after taking your medicine.

It's important to note that these are only general guidelines for managing genital herpes through diet.

Step 3: Manage Your Stress

Stress can trigger outbreaks, so it is important to manage your stress in order to stay healthy. This may mean taking breaks throughout the day or scheduling time for yourself with friends or family members. You could also try practicing yoga, meditation, deep breathing exercises, or writing in a journal when you are feeling stressed. You may also want to ask your primary care physician about taking stress relief medications if the problem becomes chronic.

Minimize your stress

People with HSV-1 are more likely to experience stress than people who do not have the virus. Research shows that having the herpes simplex virus may trigger systemic inflammation, which can increase feelings of anxiety and depression. Taking steps like those listed above for managing daily stress is one way to minimize your risk of experiencing a herpes outbreak when you're under a lot of pressure.

Sample Recipes

Below are some sample recipes that you can incorporate into your life to help manage any potential outbreaks or triggers.

Asparagus and Greens Salad with Tahini and Poppy Seed Dressing

Ingredients:

- 10 to 12 asparagus stalks, washed well and sliced into ribbons
- 5 radishes, washed well and sliced thinly
- 2 to 3 rainbow carrots, peeled and sliced thinly
- 1 handful of wild spinach
- 1 small handful of microgreens, washed well
- 1 small handful of sunflower greens, washed well
- optional: a few pieces of chive blossoms

For the dressing:

- 2 tbsp. tahini
- 1 tbsp. poppy seeds
- 1 tbsp. extra-virgin olive oil
- salt
- pepper

Instructions:

1. For the dressing, whisk ingredients together in a small bowl.
2. In a separate bowl, toss salad ingredients into the mixture.
3. Drizzle dressing on salad upon serving.

Cauliflower and Mushroom Bake

Ingredients:

- 3 cups cauliflower florets
- 1 cup fresh mushroom, chopped
- 1/2 cup red onion, chopped
- 1/3 cup green onion, chopped
- 2 garlic cloves, finely chopped
- 2 tsp. apple cider vinegar
- 2 tsp. lemon juice
- 1/2 tsp. salt
- 1/4 tsp. pepper*
- 1 tbsp. olive oil

Instructions:

1. Preheat the oven to 350°F. Lightly grease a baking pan.
2. Combine red onion, cauliflower, olive oil, garlic, mushroom, apple cider vinegar, lemon juice, salt, and pepper in a bowl. Mix well.
3. Pour the mixture into the greased baking pan.
4. Place inside the oven and bake for 45 minutes. Stir.
5. When vegetables are golden brown and tender, remove them from the oven.
6. Garnish with green onions. Serve and enjoy.

*black pepper may be substituted with white pepper

Lemon Roasted Broccoli

Ingredients:

- 1-1/2 lb. broccoli florets
- 1/3 cup shredded Parmesan cheese
- 1/4 cup olive oil
- 2 tbsps. fresh basil, chopped
- 3 tsp. minced garlic
- 1/2 – 3/4 tsp. kosher salt
- 1/2 tsp. red chili flakes
- 1/2 lemon juice and zest

Instructions:

1. Preheat the oven to 425°F.
2. Line a baking sheet with parchment paper and spread the broccoli florets.
3. Season the broccoli with basil, olive oil, garlic, kosher salt, chili flakes, lemon zest, and lemon juice.
4. Sprinkle the top with parmesan cheese then put it into the oven for 20-25 minutes or until the cheese has slightly melted.
5. Serve and enjoy while warm.

Mixed Vegetable Roast with Lemon Zest

Ingredients:

- 1-1/2 cups broccoli florets
- 1-1/2 cups cauliflower florets
- 3/4 cup red bell pepper, diced
- 3/4 cup zucchini, diced
- 2 thinly sliced cloves of garlic
- 2 tsp. lemon zest
- 1 tbsp. olive oil
- a pinch of salt
- 1 tsp. dried and crushed oregano

Instructions:

1. Preheat the oven to 425°F for 25 minutes.
2. Combine garlic and florets of broccoli and cauliflower in a baking pan.
3. Drizzle oil evenly over the vegetables. Season with salt and oregano.
4. Stir the vegetables to coat them evenly.
5. Place the pan inside the oven and roast for 10 minutes.
6. Add zucchini and bell pepper to the mix. Toss to combine.
7. Continue roasting for 10 to 15 minutes more until the vegetables turn light brown.
8. Drizzle lemon zest over vegetables and toss.
9. Serve and enjoy.

Roasted Veggies

Ingredients:

- 1/2 lb. turnips
- 1/2 lb. carrots
- 1/2 lb. parsnips
- 2 shallots, peeled
- 1/4 tsp. ground black pepper
- 1 tbsps. extra-virgin olive oil
- 6 cloves garlic
- 3/4 tsp. kosher salt
- 2 tbsp. fresh rosemary needles

Instructions:

1. First, cut vegetables into bite-sized pieces.
2. Set the oven to 400°F.
3. Mix all the ingredients in a baking dish.
4. Roast the vegetables for 25 minutes until brown and tender.
5. Toss and roast again for 20–25 minutes.
6. Serve and enjoy while hot.

Stir Fry Broccoli, Onions, and Carrots

Ingredients:

- 1 tsp. light olive oil
- 1-1/2 cups onion
- 2 cups medium-sized carrots
- 6 cups medium-sized broccoli
- 2-1/2-inch broccoli florets
- 1/4 tsp. of sea salt
- 1/2 cup of water

Instructions:

1. In a pan, heat sesame oil to medium-high heat.
2. Sauté onions. Add in carrots, broccoli, florets, and then water.
3. Season with sea salt, and cover the pan to bring to a boil.
4. Lower the heat and bring it to a simmer for 5 minutes.
5. Pour some soy sauce if needed.

Optional:

- Top some pasta or rice with stir-fried vegetables.
- Substitute other vegetables with cabbage, cauliflower, or yellow squash.
- For additional flavor, sauté 1 tbsp. minced ginger before adding carrots.

Healthy Vegetable Bowl

Ingredients:

- 1 cup of cooked brown rice
- 1 sweet potato, cut into chunks
- 1 tsp. oil
- salt and pepper
- 1 can organic chickpeas, drained
- 1-1/2 tbsp. sriracha
- 1/2 tsp. paprika
- 1/2 tsp. garlic powder
- 1 cup chopped red cabbage
- 1 cup baby spinach
- 1 avocado, sliced

Turmeric tahini sauce:

- 4 tbsp. tahini
- 4 tbsp. warm water
- 1/4 tsp. cayenne pepper
- 1/2 tsp. turmeric
- 1/2 tsp. sriracha
- salt, to taste

Instructions:

1. Preheat the oven to 180°C.
2. Place the sweet potato in a baking tray. Coat with olive oil and season it with salt. Add some pepper.

3. Pop it into the oven to roast for 35 minutes.
4. In a bowl, combine the chickpeas, sriracha, paprika, garlic powder, salt, and pepper. Mix well.
5. Heat a saucepan and transfer the chickpea mixture into it to cook for 5-10 minutes
6. In a separate saucepan, wilt the spinach slightly and season. Transfer to a bowl and repeat.
7. Place rice at the bottom of a bowl.
8. Add the spinach, sweet potato, chickpeas, red cabbage, and avocado.
9. Serve while warm.

Veggie Bowl

Ingredients:

Cauliflower Rice and Peas:

- florets from 1 pc. cauliflower
- 1 tsp. olive oil
- 1/2 onion, chopped finely
- 1 clove garlic, minced
- 1 tsp. dried thyme
- 15-oz. can kidney beans, drained
- 1/4 cup canned coconut milk

Veggies:

- 1 large sweet potato, peeled and chopped into coins
- 2 pcs. red peppers, chopped into chunks
- 1 green plantain, chopped into coins
- 1 onion, chopped roughly into wedges
- 2 pcs. zucchinis, chopped
- 1 tbsp. olive oil
- 1/2 tsp. dried thyme
- 1/2 tsp. ground allspice
- salt
- pepper
- optional: vegetable seasoning

Mango Habanero Vinaigrette:

- 1 mango, peeled and chopped roughly

- 1 clove of garlic, chopped roughly
- 1/4 small habanero pepper, chopped roughly
- 1 tbsp. red wine vinegar
- 1 tsp. Dijon mustard
- 1 tsp. olive oil
- optional: fresh cilantro, chopped

Instructions:

To make the cauliflower rice and peas:

1. Pulse a third of the florets into a food processor. Process for about 10 seconds until the florets resemble rice kernels.
2. Transfer the cauliflower rice to a large bowl.
3. Repeat until all the florets have been pulsed.
4. Heat up a teaspoon of olive oil in a sauté pan over medium heat.
5. Add the onion. Cook for about a couple of minutes.
6. Put the garlic and dried thyme. Cook for another minute.
7. Pour in the kidney beans. Stir and leave for another minute.
8. Pour in the coconut milk, followed by the cauliflower rice.
9. Cook while stirring occasionally, until the rice is slightly tender, for about 4-5 minutes. Sprinkle with salt and pepper.

10. Once done, take off the heat and set it aside. Adjust taste if necessary.

To make the grilled veggies:

1. Toss the vegetables in a bowl or on a baking sheet.
2. Drizzle with olive oil. Add in the vegetable seasoning, allspice, thyme, salt, and pepper. Toss again to coat the vegetables.
3. If using a stove, heat up a grill pan over medium-high heat. If using a barbecue grill, heat it up to medium heat.
4. Cook the veggies in batches, until they are tender and have a nice char on the outside.
5. Sweet potatoes and plantains will need to cook for about 7 minutes on each side, red pepper for about 5-6 minutes on each side, and zucchini and onions for about 3-4 minutes on each side.

To make the mango habanero vinaigrette:

1. Place all the vinaigrette ingredients into a food processor, or blender.
2. Blend until the mixture reaches a smooth consistency.

To assemble the veggie bowls:

1. Place about a cup and a half of cauliflower rice and peas into a bowl.

2. Top it off with about 2 cups of mixed veggies.
3. Drizzle the veggies with 3 tbsp. of vinaigrette. Sprinkle with fresh cilantro if desired.
4. Serve immediately and enjoy.

Healthy Zucchini Fries

Ingredients:

- 1 zucchini, cut into even strips and deseeded with a vegetable peeler
- 1 large egg
- 1/2 cup panko bread crumbs
- 1/2 cup parmesan cheese, grated
- 3/4 tsp. Italian seasoning
- 1/4 tsp. garlic powder
- pepper
- cooking spray

For yogurt dip:

- 1/2 cup yogurt
- 1/2 tsp. lemon zest
- 1 tbsp. lemon juice
- 1/8 tsp. pepper

Instructions:

1. Lightly beat the egg in a bowl.
2. In another bowl, mix the panko bread crumbs, Parmesan cheese, garlic powder, pepper, and Italian seasoning.
3. Dip the zucchini pieces into the egg. Next, put them in the crumb mixture. Coat the zucchini pieces evenly.
4. Lightly coat the air fryer basket with some oil.

5. Place half of the zucchini in the basket in one layer. Spray some oil over the zucchini pieces.
6. Arrange the remaining pieces on the top of the first layer, perpendicularly. Spray some oil over them.
7. Cook in the air fryer for 10 minutes at 400°F, or until the zucchini pieces turn golden.
8. For the yogurt dip, mix the yogurt with the lemon zest, juice, and pepper in a small bowl.
9. Serve with zucchini fries with the yogurt dip.

Avocado and Caesar Salad

Ingredients:

- 1 head romaine heart, washed
- 1 package of tempeh
- 1 small red onion, chopped
- 1/2 avocado, sliced
- sea salt
- umeboshi vinegar

Instruction:

1. Place red onions in a bowl.
2. Add a dash of sea salt and about 3 drops of umeboshi vinegar.
3. Rub the salt and vinegar mixture very gently into the onion. Do so until the color deepens. Set aside.
4. Tear apart the lettuce and place it into a bowl.
5. Add in the red onion mixture, followed by the tempeh.
6. Toss the salad lightly using a wooden spoon or with your hands.
7. Add the avocado. Toss again.
8. Drizzle a dash of umeboshi vinegar over the salad. Toss to blend the ingredients.

Cobb Salad

Ingredients:

- 1-1/2 cups quinoa
- 1 tsp. kosher salt
- 1/4 cup olive oil, plus more
- a bunch of scallions
- 3 tbsp. fresh lemon juice
- 1 avocado, cut into 1-inch pieces
- 1-pint cherry tomatoes
- 1/2 cup mint leaves
- black pepper, freshly ground
- sea salt

Instructions:

1. In a medium saucepan, add quinoa, 3 cups water, and kosher salt and leave to boil.
2. Reduce heat, cover, and simmer for 8-10 minutes, or until quinoa is soft.
3. Remove from heat and allow to sit for 15 minutes.
4. Use a fork to fluff the quinoa and transfer it to a large bowl.
5. In a small bowl, whisk olive oil and lemon juice.
6. Drizzle the mixture over the quinoa. Toss well.
7. Season it with salt and pepper. Let it cool.
8. Place a grill over medium-high heat.

9. Using a grill basket, grill scallions and tomatoes for about 6-8 minutes. Make sure to turn them occasionally, until charred in spots then remove them.
10. Transfer grilled pieces to a cutting board. Cut scallions into one-inch pieces.
11. On a platter, spoon quinoa and top with scallions, avocado, tomatoes, mint, and pistachios.
12. Drizzle with oil and sprinkle with sea salt.

Salmon and Asparagus

Ingredients:

- 2 salmon filets
- 14-oz. young potatoes
- 8 asparagus spears, trimmed and halved
- 2 handfuls cherry tomatoes
- 1 handful basil leaves
- 2 tbsp. extra-virgin olive oil
- 1 tbsp. balsamic vinegar

Instructions:

1. Heat oven to 428°F.
2. Arrange potatoes into a baking dish.
3. Drizzle potatoes with extra-virgin olive oil.
4. Roast potatoes until they have turned golden brown.
5. Place asparagus into the baking dish together with the potatoes.
6. Roast in the oven for 15 minutes.
7. Arrange cherry tomatoes and salmon among the vegetables.
8. Drizzle with balsamic vinegar and the remaining olive oil.
9. Roast until the salmon is cooked.
10. Throw in basil leaves before transferring everything to a serving dish.
11. Serve while hot.

Lemon-Baked Salmon

Ingredients:

- 2 pcs. lemons, thinly sliced
- 3 lbs. salmon filet
- kosher salt
- black pepper, freshly ground
- 6 tbsp. butter, melted, 6 tbsp.
- 2 tbsp. honey
- 3 cloves garlic, minced
- 1 tsp. thyme leaves, chopped
- 1 tsp. dried oregano
- fresh parsley, chopped, for garnish

Instructions:

1. Preheat the oven to 350°F.
2. Line a rimmed baking sheet with foil. Grease with cooking oil spray.
3. Lay lemon slices on the center of the foil.
4. Season salmon filets on both sides with kosher salt and freshly ground black pepper.
5. Place the filet on top of the lemon slices.
6. Whisk together oregano, thyme, garlic, honey, and butter in a small bowl.
7. Pour the mixture over the salmon filet.
8. Fold the foil up and around the salmon to form a packet.

9. Bake for 25 minutes or until the salmon is cooked through.
10. Switch to broil and continue cooking for 2 more minutes.
11. Garnish with chopped fresh parsley and serve hot.

Baked Salmon

Ingredients:

- 2 salmon fillets
- 6 cups of fresh spinach
- 2 tsp. coconut oil
- 1/4 tsp. garlic powder
- 1/4 tsp. turmeric
- 3 large cloves of garlic
- lemon juice
- salt
- pepper

Instructions:

1. Preheat the oven to 400°F.
2. Line a baking dish with parchment paper.
3. Marinate salmon fillets in lemon juice, coconut oil, garlic powder, turmeric, salt, and pepper.
4. Let it sit for a few minutes. This may also be done the night before to help the juices and flavor get into the salmon.
5. Once the oven is ready, bake the salmon for 15 minutes.
6. Cook some of the garlic in a pan with coconut oil.

7. Add spinach and cook until ready. Season with salt and pepper to taste.
8. Take salmon out of the oven and put spinach beside it.
9. Serve and enjoy.

Salmon Filet with Lemon and Garlic

Ingredients:

- 1 large salmon filet
- 1/4 cup fresh cilantro leaves, chopped roughly
- 4 cloves of garlic, minced
- 1 lemon
- Kosher salt, to taste
- black pepper, to taste
- Optional: 1 tbsp. butter

Instructions:

1. Preheat the oven or grill to 400°F.
2. Line a baking sheet with foil. Don't grease it.
3. Place salmon on the foil, skin side down.
4. Season the filet by squeezing lemon over it. Then, evenly sprinkle the filet with cilantro, garlic, salt, and pepper over the top.
5. Optional: Thinly slice butter and place pieces evenly over the top of the salmon.
6. For the grill, cook salmon for about 15 minutes.
7. For the oven, cook salmon for about 7 minutes, depending on its thickness.
8. Turn the oven up to broil and continue to cook for an additional 5-7 minutes, until the top is crispy.

9. Remove the salmon from the oven or grill and slide a flat spatula in between the salmon and the skin. Leave the skin to stick to the foil.
10. Serve while hot.

Roasted Broccoli and Salmon

Ingredients:

- 1-1/2 lbs. or 1 bunch of broccoli, cut into florets
- 4 tbsp. avocado oil, divided
- 1 tsp salt
- 1 tsp pepper
- 4 pcs. salmon filets, deskinned
- 1 pc. jalapeño or red Fresno chile, deseeded and sliced into thin rings
- 2 tbsp. unseasoned rice vinegar
- 2 tbsp. capers, drained

Instructions:

1. Preheat the oven to 400° F.
2. On a large, rimmed baking sheet, place the broccoli florets followed by 2 tbsp. avocado oil and season it with salt and pepper.
3. Roast the florets in the oven for 12 or 15 minutes. Toss occasionally.
4. Remove from the oven when the florets are crisp-tender and browned.
5. Gently rub the salmon filets with 1 tbsp. of the avocado oil. Season with salt and pepper.
6. Place the salmon in the middle of the baking sheet. Move the florets to the sides of the baking sheet.

7. Roast the filet for 10 to 15 minutes or until the filets turn opaque throughout.
8. In a small bowl, combine the vinegar, chile rings, and a pinch of salt. Let the mixture sit for about 10 minutes, allowing the chile rings to soften a bit.
9. Add the capers and the remaining avocado oil. Add salt and pepper to taste.
10. Drizzle chile vinaigrette over the roasted broccoli and salmon just before serving.

Smoked Salmon and Baked Eggs in Avocado

Ingredients:

- 4 oz. smoked salmon
- 8 eggs
- 4 avocados, halved and deseeded
- fresh dill
- red chili flakes
- salt
- black pepper

Instructions:

1. Preheat the oven to 425°F.
2. In preparing the avocado, make sure that the hole where the seed was can fit an egg. Carve it out more if needed.
3. Place the avocados on a baking sheet.
4. Put smoked salmon strips on each hollow.
5. Crack open an egg in a small bowl. Spoon out the yolk and the white and transfer to the avocado. Carefully eyeball how much egg the avocado can hold.
6. Sprinkle the avocado with salt and pepper.
7. Bake in the oven for about 15-20 minutes.
8. Top with dill and chili flakes upon serving.

Tuna and Veggies Wrap

Ingredients:

- 1 canned tuna
- 2 pcs. whole-grain tortillas
- 1 cup cucumber, sliced
- 1 tbsp. low-fat Italian dressing
- 1 cup carrots, julienned

Instructions:

1. Put the dressing and tuna in a bowl and mix well.
2. Arrange half of the mixture on one of the tortillas. Add half the amount of each vegetable and wrap.
3. Do the same to the remaining tortilla.

Conclusion

Although genital herpes does not have a cure, there are many actions you can take to prevent or reduce the effects of an outbreak. You can manage stress, eat right, and take medications that treat the symptoms of herpes. Following a 3-Step Plan for Managing Genital Herpes through nutrition will help improve your long-term health while reducing your risk of having an outbreak without severe side effects.

If you enjoyed this guide please leave a review. Thank you and best of luck!

References and Helpful Links

Administration, U. D. of V. A., Veterans Health. (n.d.). Va. Gov | veterans affairs [General Information]. Retrieved December 11, 2022, from https://www.publichealth.va.gov/infectiondontpassiton/womens-health-guide/stds/genital-herpes.asp.

Genital herpes | healthlink bc. (n.d.). Retrieved December 11, 2022, from https://www.healthlinkbc.ca/healthlinkbc-files/genital-herpes.

Genital herpes—Know everything about this sexually transmitted disease! (n.d.). Lybrate. Retrieved December 11, 2022, from https://www.lybrate.com/topic/genital-herpes-know-everything-about-this-sexually-transmitted-disease/fbf7c5ecf3fedc2117b2e4bd6e06d823.

Genital herpes. (n.d.). [Text]. Retrieved December 11, 2022, from https://medlineplus.gov/genitalherpes.html.

Genital herpes. (n.d.). Retrieved December 11, 2022, from https://www.palmbeachskin.com/articles/general/895933-genital-herpes.

What about diet and herpes (HSV-1 and HSV-2)? (n.d.). Retrieved December 11, 2022, from https://www.herpes.org.nz/about-herpes-questions/diet-herpes.

www.ingramcontent.com/pod-product-compliance
Lightning Source LLC
LaVergne TN
LVHW012038060526
838201LV00061B/4663